Thyroid Neuropathy and Myopathy Questions and Answers

Quality Information Exchange Between Fellow Patients

By: James M. Lowrance © 2013

TABLE OF CONTENT HYPERLINKS (click to go to each):

INTRODUCTION (pages 3 and 4)

QUESTION & ANSWER 1 (pages 5-7)

QUESTION & ANSWER 2 (pages 8-10)

QUESTION & ANSWER 3 (pages 11-13)

QUESTION & ANSWER 4 (pages 14-16)

QUESTION & ANSWER 5 (pages 17-19)

QUESTION & ANSWER 6 (pages 20-23)

About the Author (pages 25 and 25)

INTRODUCTION:

This eBook contains 6 of the best "Question and Answer" discussions that I have had with fellow thyroid myopathy and neuropathy patients, over the years (approx. 3,900 words in length). The people who asked me these questions, came to know me through the many thyroid disease books and articles I have published since year-2005. They were also aware of the fact that I was diagnosed with peripheral neuropathy and myopathy, as a result of thyroid disease and nutritional deficiencies and that I have been receiving ongoing treatment for them. While these discussions are mainly about symptoms and diagnoses of metabolic muscle and nerve diseases, treatments for them are also discussed.

For more information on treatments, see my book titled: *"Neuropathy and Myopathy in Treated Thyroid Disease"*.

Certainly patients should look to their doctors for direction and advice, first and foremost but it can bring additional comfort when one can relate to another patient who has actually "been there". Experiencing significant, negative changes in nerves and muscles of the body, can be a scary thing.

It can be very helpful to hear from someone else who has experienced the same fears and struggles, that these conditions can bring. While the information contained in the Q & A that follows, is not as extensive as one can find within a medical journal, it still touches on many of the concerns that arise within thyroid patients, who experience symptoms of chronic nerve pain and muscle weakness.

It is my hope that this general informational resource proves to be helpful and educational to those who obtain it.

- *Jim Lowrance*

QUESTION 1: I was treated for Grave's disease hyperthyroidism two years ago but after it was corrected by thyroidectomy (*thyroid gland removal*) I became hyperthyroid again, after inadvertently taking too much prescribed thyroid hormone for over a month. Is thyroid myopathy the result of hyperthyroidism, whether it occurs from being over-medicated on thyroid hormones (*dose induced thyrotoxicity*) or from an overactive thyroid gland? I'm asking this question because I'm very afraid that my overall muscle weakness means that I may have a type of muscular dystrophy. *This question was asked by a very concerned thyroid patient, who was trying to find a definitive cause for their muscle weakness, which over time had become severe enough to hinder their ability to walk more than short distances.*

ANSWER 1: I personally, was over-medicated on thyroid hormones (over-treatment thyrotoxicity) for nearly a year -- maybe more than that, on-and-off these past 10 years of my own hormone replacement therapy. I feel however that my development of myopathy, resulted from a phase of hyperthyroidism I experienced early into my autoimmune hypothyroid disease (Hashimoto's thyroiditis). However, I feel that thyroid patients can experience myopathy, even if they never see hyperthyroidism from over-treatment or from any other cause.

I say this because "metabolic myopathies", can happen with any disease affecting metabolism (e.g. diabetes, adrenal insufficiency or hyper-function and liver disease).

I can understand your concern, I felt scared as well however, it's still very likely a manifestation of your thyroid disease and not a muscular dystrophy type disease, as you expressed concern about. Even if it were this type of disease however (please know that I'm only adding this because I know you feel scared), those diseases affecting adults, don't usually become life threatening before old age and people with them usually live normal lifespans. There's only one condition in the muscle disease category that I know of, that is life-threatening to adults and that's "ALS" (Lou Gehrig's Disease – very rare) and yours does not at all manifest like that one. One would not have an overall muscle weakness, as you described having but they would see severe atrophy in one limb (muscle wasting/shrinkage) before ALS would be suspected -- usually in a leg.

I'm so sorry about your struggle with the muscle weakness. My myopathy also makes it difficult to walk moderate and long distances at times but there hasn't been any overall, significant worsening of mine, beyond my first year of hypothyroid treatment.

I now don't believe mine was from any over-treatment with thyroid hormone. As I stated previously regarding thyroid myopathy in general, I believe mine to be mainly from thyroid disease itself -- the "autoimmunity" aspect. That may sound like a strange statement but I feel that the "antibodies" involved in autoimmune thyroid diseases, can potentially cause we thyroid patients, certain types of symptoms apart from where our thyroid hormones are (even when in optimal ranges).

It is possible for treated **hypo**thyroid patients (those with under-active thyroid glands and no thyrotoxicity) to experience chronic nerve and muscle problems as well but less commonly than **hyper**thyroid patients. I think in your case though, with your relating to me that it has only been 5 months since your hyperthyroidism was corrected, that you could still see some improvement -- that's very possible. Of course I'm a layperson and I can only make an educated guess, based on my extensive search and research in these areas.

I do wish you the best with your definitive diagnosis and with your treatments and be sure to follow your doctor's treatment instructions, carefully.

QUESTION 2: My doctor has run a number of tests, to determine if my muscle weakness has another cause apart from my thyroid disease such as blood tests for anemia and diabetes but no other causes have yet been found. Does your thyroid myopathy cause you muscle-soreness as mine does and do you feel that a muscle biopsy test should be ordered to better evaluate this condition?

ANSWER 2: Yes, at times when my myopathy is flaring worse, I feel muscle soreness very easily with any activity. If I may say, I wonder if you have yet to be worked up well enough on blood tests, such as your "CK" level (Creatine Kinase)? More of this enzyme leaks from the muscles, into the bloodstream, if actual muscle damage is occurring, such as with actual neuromuscular diseases. You did say that your muscles don't seem to be having atrophy in them (wasting, shrinking), so it's possible that these type blood tests are unwarranted. I also wonder if they tested your major vitamin levels, especially B12 and D? If not, these tests would be well worth being ordered by your doctor.

Regarding the muscle biopsy test you asked about, I haven't personally had one performed but I may actually ask my doctor to refer me for one soon.

9

I have wondered, what category of severeness my own thyroid myopathy would fall under at this point (e.g. mild, moderate or severe). I have Chronic Fatigue Syndrome as well but that has more to do with a feeling of tiredness and not necessarily weakness in the muscles, although some CFS patients do have a type of muscle weakness as well, as part of their symptoms.

It's very concerning when you have something, like you and I have but it remains a mystery as to a definitive reason for it. I'm sure there is a statistic somewhere showing that a percent of myopathy, never has a cause found for it, just as 1/3 of peripheral neuropathy patients have no cause found for their damaged nerves (idiopathic - unknown).

In my case, I also now have diabetes which caused me to be very angry at myself for allowing my weight-gain to contribute to it, which can also contribute further to my nerve and muscle issues. However, with my thyroid disease and certain medications I take, the weight gain is common and more difficult to control. I am currently working on a weight loss plan however, which can help to improve my myopathy symptoms significantly, by simply relieving the added stress to them.

Since I have mentioned medications, let me also point out that neither myopathy nor peripheral neuropathy, that are caused by metabolic diseases including thyroid disorders, have treatments available that will completely reverse them. They can however, be slowed down and possibly halted by correcting these underlying medical conditions that cause them. Otherwise, the only treatments doctors can offer, are medications that help to control the symptoms of them. This would include those prescribed to control nerve pain in peripheral neuropathy patients and those that serve as muscle relaxers, should muscle tension or spasms occur in certain myopathy patients.

Physical therapies can help with these conditions as well and with some types of mono-neuropathies, such as carpal tunnel and other single nerve entrapments, physical therapy can actually rescue a blocked/pinched nerve. Poly-neuropathies (many nerves affected), usually indicate that irreversible damage has occurred to the affected nerves and some peripheral neuropathies affect the "motor nerves" as well, causing weakness to muscles. This is why these conditions often run together and why doctors have the task of determining whether or not there is damaged nerve involvement in cases of myopathy.

I hope my general but somewhat detailed response was of help to you.

QUESTION 3: Other than thyroid tests and extensive blood testing I have had done in regard to my thyroid myopathy, should I have a repeat EMG (my first one was 5 months ago) or a QSART test done, to further evaluate my muscle-weakness (or other tests you might suggest)? *Note: An EMG is an "Electromyography", which records the electrical activity produced by skeletal muscles and a QSART is a "Quantitative Sudomotor Axon Reflex Test", which measures the autonomic nerves that control sweating, and is useful in assessing autonomic nervous system disorders.*

ANSWER 3: Your thyroid labs which you shared with me, do look good. It's also good that you had the full battery of blood testing done. I don't know if an EMG would be worthwhile, so soon after you having the first one done. Was your first one in normal ranges? If so, it's very unlikely they would show any difference after only 5 months. The same true if they <u>were not</u> all normal. You might ask your doctor what he/she would think about ordering you a muscle biopsy. I had a tissue biopsy done on one leg (a small fiber nerve biopsy) and they had to do it twice. It was not bad at all and I cannot find the two hole punch scars from it anymore. I suspect that a muscle biopsy, which they take from the thigh area of the leg, wouldn't be much worse.

I'm like you -- I want to have one performed as well, simply to round out and follow up on my own diagnosis but I'm not completely sure what to expect invasive-wise.

I did have peripheral neuropathy identified with my EMG test but my doctor didn't feel that it was the cause of my muscle weakness because sensory nerves are usually involved first, long before motor nerves are affected by peripheral neuropathy (those that control muscle movement and strength).

I do have pain with mine but never severe. I have also not had the QSART done but I did a quick search and see that it is a test for monitoring nerves to sweat glands. That's interesting and makes me wonder why my doctor didn't order that one for me originally, in light of the fact that I do experience some involuntary nervous system dysfunction.

I become dizzy when I first stand up, which means my blood pressure takes longer than normal to regulate when my body position changes (orthostatic hypo-tension). This can be, but is not always a sign that autonomic neuropathy is occurring. Possibly my doctor felt my small fiber tissue biopsy was sufficient, which showed only mild "sensory nerve" damage.

13

You might consider discussing the QSART one with your doctor, if you seem to be experiencing any problems with your involuntary body functions, which are mainly controlled by autonomic nerves (e.g. heart rate, breathing, bowel function, etc...). Best wishes with it and let me know how it goes!

QUESTION 4: I am a thyroid patient with body pain and weakness and my doctor has conducted two different EMG tests on me, only a few months apart, with the second one showing fast progression of my (so far), mild thyroid myopathy and neuropathy. With that last test being several months ago and with my fast-onset symptoms showing no improvement, what further tests should I discuss having done, with my doctor – maybe a new EMG? *Typical nerve pain and muscle weakness symptoms were described to me by this 42 year old fellow patient, when they submitted their question to me and they described their thyroid disease, as being the temporary, thyroid-inflammatory condition known as "Silent thyroiditis".*

ANSWER 4: Your circumstance is kind of extraordinary because from the information you related, it sounds like your nerve changes did have a fast onset. Possibly another EMG would be the thing you need right now, in light of the fact that some abnormalities were found the other times you had these done, several months ago and only a few months apart. I mention this because there is a condition called "Chronic Inflammatory Demyelinating Polyneuropathy" (CIDP), which usually follows a viral infection and this one can develop rapidly but is easily and almost always successfully treatable.

It usually first manifests in one limb of the body, most often in the affected person's hand, wrist or foot. In addition to CIDP, there are other types of neuropathy and myopathy, that can onset rapidly but these are all quite rare.

In my own case of somewhat elusive muscle weakness, my own neurologist ordered a lumbar puncture (spinal fluid tap), to test me for Multiple Sclerosis, Lyme disease and other diseases that can be revealed in spinal fluid. Mine was negative for these but I felt somewhat sick after getting that test done! I was head-achy and nauseous for nearly a month on and off after getting the procedure done. Still, I was glad to get it past me for some peace of mind.

I'm actually wondering if you retained the mild myopathy, due to your temporary thyroid disease -- and as you said, an EMG, might reveal whether or not any muscle or nerve damage, has progressed or regressed. When I searched reputable medical sites sometime ago, I was surprised at what they considered to be "mild" and "moderate" myopathies. The symptoms you described, would be in the milder category. The more severe types do cause people to be in wheelchairs etc... My feelings are that while yours hasn't corrected, that it will likely remain mild.

I say that because you know what caused it -- the Silent Thyroiditis, and that it has been resolved. It can't continue to cause further damage to your nerves. You could still see some improvement as well and some doctors suggest giving a full year for myopathy from a temporary thyroiditis to resolve. For peace of mind, you could discuss a new EMG with your doctor.

I want to add that if by chance they diagnosed you with MS (one of the concerns you expressed in the main body of your letter), which is very unlikely because yours sounds like common metabolic myopathy, that this also is not a death sentence. Most MS patients, as well as myopathy patients (like you and me), live normal lifespans, although with symptom-struggles along the way. I honestly feel that your myopathy was from the thyroiditis and likely will only worsen some with age (nerves also degrade naturally over time). Do what you can to keep your body healthy and strong (that's what I'm doing) and you may not see any significant problems, until you're in your 60s or 70s.

QUESTION 5: I have experienced vague neuropathy symptoms for more than 3 years but after experiencing sub-acute thyroiditis (painful, temporary thyroid inflammation), I was left with more serious nerve and muscle symptoms, plus some hyperthyroid symptoms. Since it has been 5 months since my illness, with no improvements, should I opt for nerve function testing? *NOTE: This fellow patient is also a close friend of mine and he provided me copies of his doctor's reports, to help me provide a general, layperson answer to his question.*

ANSWER 5: Did your sub-acute thyroiditis present with hyperthyroidism, following hypothyroidism or was it the reverse? I know that sounds like a strange question but most people who experience this condition, see a short term phase of hyperthyroidism and possibly a phase of hypothyroidism, afterward. In some cases, the hypothyroidism becomes permanent, requiring lifelong treatment. Were you treated with an "anti-thyroid drug" (to lower thyroid hormones) or were you given thyroid hormones for a period of time? In your medical reports, the doctor states that the mild myopathy is likely from "the hypothyroidism". I think your frustration is not knowing if it is caused only by the thyroiditis and related, short-term thyroid hormone imbalances or from something else.

You said you felt some vague symptoms for over 3 years and a significant increase in them, after experiencing the painful, temporary goiter. However, you've only been five months, post thyroiditis, so you could still see improvements in your nerves and muscles, that is yet to come, given another few months. Your doctor also informed you that your thyroid disease did not become a permanent type. Your idea that the doctor do an EMG test on you (nerve testing), might be a good one and might offer you peace of mind, by providing you more answers. He did mention a suspicion of "Cushings disease" in your medical test reports, which is a term for the syndrome of having too much adrenal cortisol hormone in your system, so possibly they should do a blood cortisol blood draw, if not already done.

You'll be surprised to read this but the "vitamin E" blood test they did for you, was done for me, and mine came back at "0.4" -- less than a half-point in my body, with normal range being "5.0 to 16.0"! This deficiency may be a major factor in my own development of peripheral neuropathy. This is one of the vitamins I'm on permanent regimen to take, along with vitamin D, which I was also deficient on and vitamin B12, which I had low-normal - "insufficient" levels of. All of these deficiencies can result in neuropathy and myopathy type symptoms.

Your vitamin levels were apparently all okay, which helps you to eliminate, just that many more possibilities as a cause of your symptoms.

That EMG, might be the best way to know where the myopathy is at (mild, moderate or severe) but I'm betting it would still show mild, based on the description of symptoms you provided me. Still, it might give you some comfort if they can tell that it's not progressing and possibly even regressing. I hope that's the case for you.

QUESTION 6: I experienced an episode of Silent Thyroiditis, after giving birth and mine came with a period of strong hyperthyroidism, that lasted about 3 weeks. My doctor who is an endocrinologist, says I'm negative for thyroid antibodies. The thyroiditis got better but it left me with weakened muscles and strong muscle burn feelings with any exercise, nearly 6 months later. My doctor also told me that this is myopathy and that it should get better over a year's period of time and with precautionary thyroid blood retesting, physical therapy and exercise. Do you think he is right in saying that my weak muscles are from the hyperthyroid spell and that the follow up suggestions will really help?

ANSWER 6: I really do believe yours is from the thyrotoxic period you went through (hyperthyroidism), with your Silent Thyroiditis. Interestingly, I went through a phase of hyperthyroidism, early into my Hashimoto's thyroiditis (a permanent disease of hypothyroidism), which is fairly common with that disease and it caused me muscle weakness, that I experience to this day. You were fortunate that yours **wasn't** the sub-acute type of thyroiditis, which is very painful in the thyroid area. It is also fortunate that you were not left with permanent thyroid disease.

The temporary types of thyroiditis, usually happen with upper respiratory viruses that settle into the thyroid gland or following pregnancies. Still, you obviously went through a hyperthyroid phase and yours may have resolved without transitioning into a phase of hypothyroidism (this is why your doctor is still blood retesting you, to make sure).

My own myopathy, is almost certainly in the mild category, just as they placed yours in. I don't have quite as much of the muscle-burn feeling as you do but I most definitely feel my muscles giving out on me, when I use them for anything even moderately strenuous (probably evenly mildly strenuous). I absolutely didn't experience the muscle weakness before having Hashimoto's disease and as a man who was trying to make a living and having strenuous work to do, it was devastating to me for this condition to come on my body. I'm now not stressing as much about it as I did when I first began experiencing it. For one thing, I achieved getting Social Security Disability benefits, which helps greatly with my medical expenses but also because I've simply adjusted better to my myopathy. I suppose I came to accept it, as time went by. You likely went through a slightly more severe hyperthyroid phase than I did.

However, with you not being found positive for thyroid antibodies - "autoimmunity" (permanent thyroid disease), yours can still improve slowly over time, as your doctor informed you.

I really believe you have the answer -- the thyroiditis that caused you the thyrotoxicity, is the culprit for your muscle symptoms. It's simply too coincidental for the myopathy to have followed your thyroiditis, for it not to be the cause. The opinion of an endocrinologist should be very reliable because they see patients with metabolic myopathies, commonly. You asked me if you should do the follow ups your doctor is suggesting, which includes more testing and physical therapy. With it being your health, you have to always err on the side of caution. That would be my advice but mostly that you should follow those gut feelings regarding your doctor's referrals to physical therapies (in the vast majority of cases, they help a great deal). The great concern you have, tells me that you don't feel you have had everything done yet, to completely satisfy your diagnosis or plan of action to take for it. Suggestions for consideration, are now being offered to you by your doctor

You also asked me if physical therapy and exercise can help to reverse the symptoms you are experiencing.

I do believe you could reverse the effects of it with practices that include exercise. I remember reading other myopathy patient's attest to seeing theirs improve, simply by gradually strengthening their bodies. Sites that list treatments for myopathy, will include "exercise" in their lists but they usually advise patient to make sure it is done safely, carefully and within tolerance levels, because overdoing with exercise can cause muscle strain and soreness.

The physical therapy will be specialized to your needs and will also help you, especially when combined with an exercise plan, for restoring a better quality of life to you.

(END)

About the Author:

I am a husband, father, grandfather and lifetime contract salesman, with experience in health writing that began in 2004. I completed theological studies with Liberty University in 1996. I formerly served as editor and forum moderator of Thyroid Health for a major multi-topic content site and as a general health writer for another, where I achieved Editor's Choice Awards for my articles on health subjects.

In 2003 I was diagnosed with hypothyroidism; "Hashimoto's thyroiditis" being the cause. This autoimmune form of thyroid disease that causes destruction of the thyroid gland resulted in my also developing "Chronic Fatigue Syndrome", due to a compromised immune system with severe co-morbid "Adrenal Fatigue".

I also suffered severe anxiety symptoms, including panic attacks early into the onset of Hashimoto's thyroiditis (Hashitoxicosis). A common, benign heart murmur I was diagnosed with in my teens called "Mitral Valve Prolapse", also worsened in severity of symptoms, with the development of these other health disorders.

My eventual receiving of diagnoses was a difficult process with proper diagnostic testing not being ordered by the first doctors I sought treatment from. These types of issues were inspiration for me to become proactive in my own health care and to self-educate myself on these health disorders, which I have done extensively since 2003.

I now enjoy sharing this information with other patients experiencing my same health disorders.

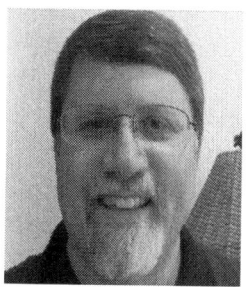